OSTEOARTHRITIS DIET COOKBOOK

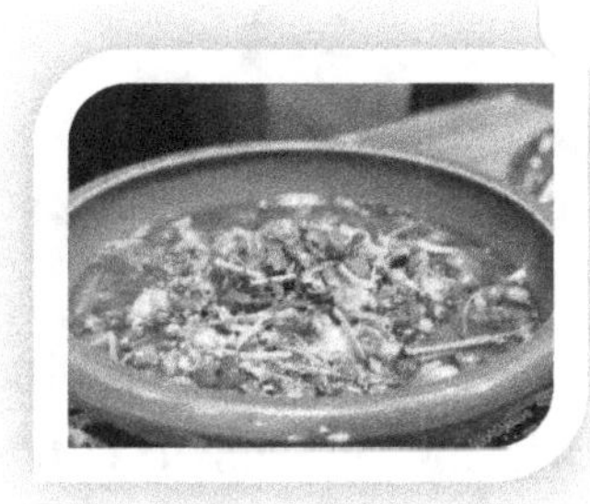

Nutrition Guide with Anti-inflammatory and Flavorful   Recipes for joint relief

DR.CATHERINE THOMAS

TABLE OF CONTENT

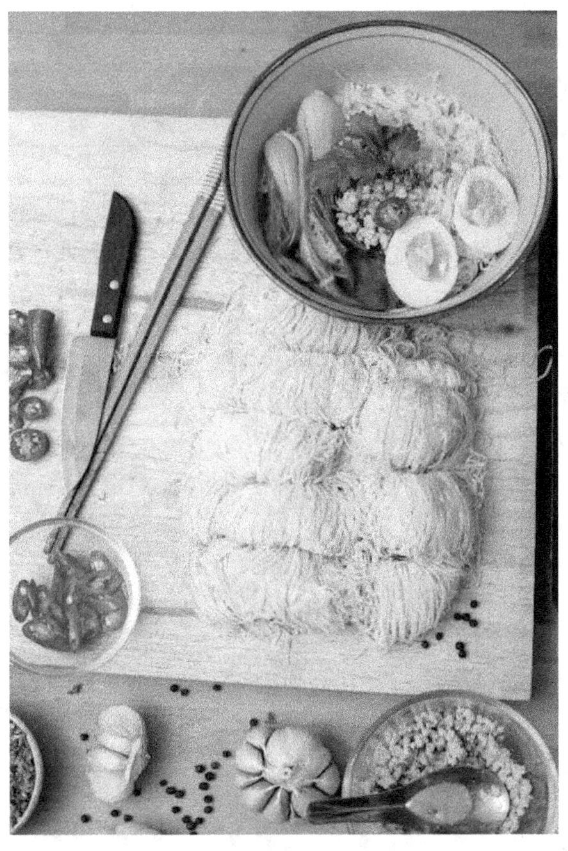

INTRODUCTION

Welcome to the **Osteoarthritis Recipe Cookbook**, your comprehensive guide to nourishing your body and alleviating joint pain through the power of food. I am **Dr. Catherine Thomas**, a dedicated nutritionist with years of experience helping individuals transform their lives through diet and lifestyle changes. This cookbook is born from my passion for promoting wellness and my commitment to providing you with the tools to lead a healthier, more vibrant life.

Osteoarthritis is a journey filled with challenges, but it is also one where informed choices can make a significant difference. I have witnessed firsthand how the right nutrition can empower individuals to take control of their health, reduce inflammation, and improve their quality of life. This book is a culmination of my professional insights, personal experiences, and the latest scientific research on the anti-inflammatory benefits of food.

Inside these pages, you will find more than just recipes; you will discover a pathway to reclaiming your vitality. Each recipe is thoughtfully designed to be both nutritious and delicious, ensuring that you never have to sacrifice flavor for health.

Whether you are seeking to soothe aching joints, increase your energy levels, or simply enjoy wholesome meals, this cookbook is here to guide you every step of the way.

The recipes within are crafted to suit a variety of tastes and dietary needs, making it easy for everyone to embrace a healthier lifestyle. From hearty breakfasts that kickstart your day to comforting dinners that help you unwind, every meal is an opportunity to nurture your body and soul.

My hope is that this cookbook will inspire you to see food not just as sustenance, but as a powerful ally in your journey toward better health. Together, we can embark on this path of healing, one delicious bite at a time.

With warmth and well wishes,

Dr. Catherine Thomas

PART 1

Understanding Osteoarthritis

Osteoarthritis (OA) is the most common form of arthritis, affecting millions of people worldwide. It is a degenerative joint disease characterized by the breakdown of cartilage, which is the smooth, protective tissue at the ends of bones. This breakdown leads to pain, swelling, and reduced motion in the joints. Understanding OA involves exploring its types, causes, symptoms, and preventive measures.

Types of Osteoarthritis

There are primarily two types of osteoarthritis:

1. **Primary Osteoarthritis:** This is the most common form and occurs as a result of aging. It is often referred to as "wear-and-tear" arthritis because it typically develops over many years. The joints most commonly affected by primary OA are the hands, knees, hips, and spine.

2. **Secondary Osteoarthritis:** This type occurs due to a specific cause or condition, such as an injury, obesity, genetics, or other medical

conditions like rheumatoid arthritis or gout. Secondary OA can develop at any age and is often localized to joints that have been previously damaged or subjected to unusual stress.

Causes of Osteoarthritis

The exact cause of osteoarthritis is multifactorial and can vary from person to person. Several factors contribute to the development of OA:

1. **Age:** The risk of developing osteoarthritis increases with age, as the cumulative wear and tear on joints take a toll over time.

2. **Joint Injury:** Previous injuries to a joint, such as fractures or ligament tears, can increase the likelihood of developing OA in that joint.

3. **Genetics:** There is evidence to suggest that OA can run in families. Certain genetic factors can make a person more susceptible to developing the disease.

4. **Obesity:** Excess body weight puts additional stress on weight-bearing joints, particularly the knees and hips, accelerating the breakdown of cartilage.

5. **Repetitive Stress:** Occupations or activities that involve repetitive motions or stress on particular joints can lead to OA. For example, athletes or workers who frequently kneel, squat, or lift heavy objects are at higher risk.

6. **Bone Deformities:** Some people are born with malformed joints or defective cartilage, which can increase the risk of OA.

7. **Metabolic Diseases:** Conditions like diabetes and hemochromatosis (a disorder that causes the body to absorb too much iron) can increase the risk of OA.

Symptoms of Osteoarthritis

The symptoms of osteoarthritis can vary depending on the severity and the joints affected. Common symptoms include:

1. **Pain:** Joint pain during or after movement is the most common symptom of OA. Pain may also be present at rest or during periods of inactivity.

2. **Stiffness:** Joint stiffness, particularly upon waking up in the morning or after periods of inactivity, is another hallmark of OA. This stiffness usually improves with movement.

3. **Tenderness:** The joint may feel tender when light pressure is applied.

4. **Loss of Flexibility:** OA can reduce the range of motion in affected joints, making it difficult to perform everyday tasks.

5. **Grating Sensation:** You may feel or hear a grating or crackling sensation when moving the joint.

6. **Bone Spurs:** These are extra bits of bone that can form around the affected joint, causing lumps that can be felt under the skin.

7. **Swelling:** Soft tissue inflammation around the joint can lead to swelling and warmth.

Preventive Measures for Osteoarthritis

While osteoarthritis cannot be completely prevented, there are several measures that can reduce the risk and slow its progression:

1. **Maintain a Healthy Weight:** Keeping your weight within a healthy range reduces stress on weight-bearing joints like the knees and hips. Even a small amount of weight loss can significantly reduce the risk of OA.

2. **Stay Active:** Regular physical activity strengthens the muscles around the joints, helping to support and protect them. Low-impact exercises such as swimming, cycling, and walking are particularly beneficial.

3. **Protect Your Joints:** Avoid activities that place excessive stress on your joints. Use proper techniques when lifting heavy objects and take breaks to avoid repetitive stress.

4. **Eat a Balanced Diet:** A diet rich in fruits, vegetables, lean proteins, and whole grains can help maintain overall health and reduce inflammation. Omega-3 fatty acids, found in fish and flaxseed, have anti-inflammatory properties.

5. **Stay Hydrated:** Drinking plenty of water helps keep your joints lubricated and supports overall joint health.

6. **Wear Proper Footwear:** Supportive shoes can help reduce stress on your knees and hips.

Avoid high heels and opt for shoes with good arch support and cushioning.

7. **Strengthen Your Muscles:** Strong muscles around the joints provide better support and reduce the risk of injury. Focus on exercises that strengthen the muscles of the legs, hips, and core.

8. **Flexibility and Balance Training:** Stretching exercises and activities that improve balance, such as yoga and tai chi, can enhance joint flexibility and prevent falls.

9. **Avoid Injury:** Take precautions to avoid joint injuries. Use protective gear during sports, practice safe techniques, and be mindful of your body's limits.

10. **Regular Check-ups:** Regular visits to your healthcare provider can help monitor joint health and detect early signs of osteoarthritis. Early intervention can slow the progression of the disease.

While osteoarthritis cannot be entirely prevented, adopting a healthy lifestyle, maintaining an optimal weight, and protecting your joints can significantly reduce the risk and impact of this debilitating disease.

PART 2

Foods to Eat and Avoid for Optimal Health with Osteoarthritis

Managing osteoarthritis (OA) through diet involves focusing on foods that reduce inflammation and support joint health while avoiding those that can exacerbate symptoms. Here's a guide to the best and worst foods for an osteoarthritis-friendly diet.

Foods to Eat

1. **Fatty Fish:** Rich in omega-3 fatty acids, fish like salmon, mackerel, and sardines have potent anti-inflammatory properties. Omega-3s help reduce joint pain and stiffness.

2. **Fruits and Vegetables:** Colorful fruits and vegetables are packed with antioxidants, vitamins, and minerals that fight inflammation. Berries, cherries, spinach, kale, and broccoli are particularly beneficial.

3. **Whole Grains:** Whole grains like brown rice, quinoa, and whole wheat are high in fiber,

which can help reduce inflammation. They also provide sustained energy and aid in weight management.

4. **Nuts and Seeds:** Almonds, walnuts, flaxseeds, and chia seeds are excellent sources of healthy fats and antioxidants. They help reduce inflammation and provide essential nutrients for joint health.

5. **Olive Oil:** Extra virgin olive oil contains oleocanthal, a compound with anti-inflammatory effects similar to ibuprofen. Use it as a primary cooking oil to support joint health.

6. **Lean Proteins:** Chicken, turkey, and plant-based proteins like beans and lentils provide the necessary building blocks for muscle repair without adding excessive fat. Strong muscles support and protect joints.

7. **Dairy:** Low-fat dairy products such as yogurt, milk, and cheese provide calcium and vitamin D, essential for bone health. These nutrients help maintain strong bones, which are crucial for joint support.

8. **Green Tea:** Rich in polyphenols and antioxidants, green tea can help reduce inflammation and slow cartilage damage.

1. **Sugary Foods and Beverages:** High sugar intake can increase inflammation and contribute to weight gain, putting extra stress on joints. Avoid sodas, candy, and other sugary snacks.

2. **Refined Carbohydrates:** White bread, pastries, and other refined carbs can spike blood sugar levels and increase inflammation. Opt for whole grains instead.

3. **Fried and Processed Foods:** These foods are often high in unhealthy fats and additives that can trigger inflammation. Avoid fried foods, fast food, and processed snacks.

4. **Red and Processed Meats:** These meats can be high in saturated fats and advanced glycation end products (AGEs), which promote inflammation. Limit consumption of beef, pork, and processed meats like sausages and hot dogs.

5. **Excessive Alcohol:** High alcohol consumption can increase inflammation and negatively impact overall health. If you drink, do so in moderation.

6. **High-Sodium Foods:** Excessive salt can lead to water retention and increase joint swelling.

Reduce intake of salty snacks, canned soups, and processed foods.

Adopting an osteoarthritis-friendly diet means focusing on anti-inflammatory foods that support overall health and joint function while avoiding those that can worsen inflammation and pain. By making mindful food choices, individuals with osteoarthritis can improve their quality of life, reduce symptoms, and achieve optimal health.

14 Day Meal Plan

Breakfast:

Greek yogurt with mixed berries and a drizzle of honey

Lunch:

Quinoa salad with chickpeas, cherry tomatoes, cucumber, and a lemon-tahini dressing

Snack:

Apple slices with almond butter

Dinner:

Baked salmon with steamed broccoli and sweet potato

Breakfast:

Overnight oats with chia seeds, almond milk, and sliced bananas

Lunch:

Turkey and avocado wrap with whole wheat tortilla, spinach, and hummus

Snack:

Carrot sticks with guacamole

Dinner:

Grilled chicken breast with quinoa and roasted vegetables (bell peppers, zucchini, and carrots)

Breakfast:

Smoothie with spinach, pineapple, banana, and flaxseed

Lunch:

Lentil soup with a side of mixed greens salad

Snack:

Handful of walnuts and a pear

Dinner:

Stir-fry with tofu, broccoli, snap peas, and brown rice

Breakfast:

Scrambled eggs with spinach and whole grain toast

Lunch:

Chickpea and avocado salad with cherry tomatoes and a balsamic vinaigrette

Snack:

Blueberries and a small handful of almonds

Dinner:

Baked cod with quinoa and steamed asparagus

Breakfast:

Whole grain pancakes with fresh berries and a dollop of Greek yogurt

Lunch:

Quinoa and black bean bowl with corn, avocado, and salsa

Snack:

Cucumber slices with hummus

Dinner:

Grilled shrimp with brown rice and roasted Brussels sprouts

Breakfast:

Smoothie bowl with mixed berries, chia seeds, and granola

Lunch:

Spinach and kale salad with grilled chicken, walnuts, and an apple cider vinaigrette

Snack:

Sliced bell peppers with tzatziki

Dinner:

Turkey chili with kidney beans, tomatoes, and spices

Breakfast:

Oatmeal with almond butter, banana slices, and a sprinkle of cinnamon

Lunch:

Tuna salad with mixed greens, cherry tomatoes, and olive oil dressing

Snack:

Fresh orange and a handful of pistachios

Dinner:

Baked chicken with wild rice and roasted carrots

Breakfast:

Smoothie with kale, mango, banana, and chia seeds

Lunch:

Quinoa and roasted vegetable salad with a lemon-tahini dressing

Snack:

Pear slices with cheese cubes

Dinner:

Grilled salmon with mashed sweet potatoes and steamed green beans

Breakfast:

Whole grain toast with avocado and poached eggs

Lunch:

Lentil and vegetable stew with a side of mixed greens salad

Snack:

Apple slices with almond butter

Dinner:

Stir-fry with chicken, bell peppers, broccoli, and brown rice

Breakfast:

Greek yogurt with mixed berries and honey

Lunch:

Spinach and quinoa salad with chickpeas, cucumbers, and a lemon vinaigrette

Snack:

Carrot sticks with hummus

Dinner:

Baked cod with quinoa and roasted Brussels sprouts

Breakfast:

Smoothie with spinach, pineapple, banana, and flaxseed

Lunch:

Turkey and avocado wrap with whole wheat tortilla, spinach, and hummus

Snack:

Handful of walnuts and a pear

Dinner:

Grilled shrimp with brown rice and roasted vegetables

Breakfast:

Scrambled eggs with spinach and whole grain toast

Lunch:

Chickpea and avocado salad with cherry tomatoes and a balsamic vinaigrette

Snack:

Blueberries and a small handful of almonds

Dinner:

Baked salmon with quinoa and steamed broccoli

Breakfast:

Whole grain pancakes with fresh berries and Greek yogurt

Lunch:

Quinoa and black bean bowl with corn, avocado, and salsa

Snack:

Cucumber slices with hummus

Dinner:

Grilled chicken with wild rice and roasted carrots

Breakfast:

Smoothie bowl with mixed berries, chia seeds, and granola

Lunch:

Spinach and kale salad with grilled chicken, walnuts, and an apple cider vinaigrette

Snack:

Sliced bell peppers with tzatziki

Dinner:

Turkey chili with kidney beans, tomatoes, and spice

PART 3

Greek Yogurt with Mixed Berries

Ingredients:

1 cup Greek yogurt (plain, non-fat)

1/2 cup mixed berries (blueberries, strawberries, raspberries)

1 tbsp honey

1 tbsp chia seeds

Preparation:

1. Place Greek yogurt in a bowl.

2. Top with mixed berries.

3. Drizzle honey over the berries.

4. Sprinkle chia seeds on top.

Nutritional Value:

Calories: 220

Protein: 20g

Fat: 5g

Carbohydrates: 30g

Fiber: 6g   **Cooking Time: 5 minutes**

Overnight Oats with Almonds and Bananas

Ingredients:

1/2 cup rolled oats

1/2 cup almond milk

1/2 banana, sliced

1 tbsp almond butter

1 tbsp chia seeds

1 tsp honey

Preparation:

1. In a jar, combine rolled oats, almond milk, almond butter, chia seeds, and honey.

2. Stir well, cover, and refrigerate overnight.

3. In the morning, top with banana slices.

Nutritional Value:

Calories: 350

Protein: 10g

Fat: 15g

Carbohydrates: 45g

Fiber: 8g

Cooking Time: 10 minutes (plus overnight refrigeration)

Spinach and Feta Omelette

Ingredients:

2 large eggs

1/2 cup fresh spinach, chopped

1/4 cup feta cheese, crumbled

1 tbsp olive oil

Salt and pepper to taste

Preparation:

1. Whisk eggs with salt and pepper.

2. Heat olive oil in a non-stick pan over medium heat.

3. Pour in the eggs and cook until they begin to set.

4. Add spinach and feta cheese to one side of the omelette.

5. Fold the omelette in half and cook for another minute.

Nutritional Value:

Calories: 250

Protein: 18g

Fat: 20g

Carbohydrates: 3g

Fiber: 1g   **Cooking Time: 10 minutes**

Smoothie Bowl with Berries and Granola

Ingredients:

1 cup frozen mixed berries

1/2 banana

1/2 cup almond milk

1/4 cup granola

1 tbsp chia seeds

Preparation:

1. Blend frozen berries, banana, and almond milk until smooth.

2. Pour into a bowl.

3. Top with granola and chia seeds.

Nutritional Value:

Calories: 300

Protein: 6g

Fat: 10g

Carbohydrates: 50g

Fiber: 8g   **Cooking Time: 10 minutes**

Whole Grain Pancakes with Fresh Berries

Ingredients:

1 cup whole grain pancake mix

3/4 cup water

1/2 cup fresh berries

1 tbsp honey

1 tbsp chia seeds

Preparation:

1. Mix pancake mix and water until smooth.

2. Heat a non-stick pan over medium heat.

3. Pour batter into the pan to form pancakes.

4. Cook until bubbles form, then flip and cook until golden brown.

5. Top with fresh berries, honey, and chia seeds.

Nutritional Value:

Calories: 320

Protein: 8g

Fat: 6g

Carbohydrates: 60g

Fiber: 10g   **Cooking Time: 15 minutes**

Avocado Toast with Poached Eggs

Ingredients:

1 slice whole grain bread

1/2 avocado, mashed

1 large egg

1 tbsp vinegar

Salt and pepper to taste

Preparation:

1. Toast the bread.

2. Spread mashed avocado on the toast.

3. Boil water with vinegar, then reduce to a simmer.

4. Crack the egg into a small bowl, then gently slide it into the water.

5. Poach for 3-4 minutes, then remove with a slotted spoon and place on toast.

6. Season with salt and pepper.

Nutritional Value:

Calories: 280

Protein: 10g

Fat: 20g

Carbohydrates: 20g

Fiber: 7g

Cooking Time: 10 minutes

Quinoa Breakfast Bowl with Almonds and Fruit

Ingredients:

1/2 cup cooked quinoa

1/4 cup almond milk

1/2 apple, diced

1 tbsp almonds, sliced

1 tsp honey

1/4 tsp cinnamon

Preparation:

1. Combine cooked quinoa and almond milk in a bowl.

2. Top with diced apple, sliced almonds, honey, and cinnamon.

Nutritional Value:

Calories: 280

Protein: 8g

Fat: 9g

Carbohydrates: 42g

Fiber: 6g   **Cooking Time: 10 minutes**

Chia Seed Pudding with Blueberries

Ingredients:

1/4 cup chia seeds

1 cup almond milk

1 tbsp honey

1/2 cup blueberries

Preparation:

1. Mix chia seeds, almond milk, and honey in a bowl.

2. Refrigerate overnight.

3. Top with blueberries before serving.

Nutritional Value:

Calories: 300

Protein: 8g

Fat: 15g

Carbohydrates: 38g

Fiber: 16g

Cooking Time: 10 minutes (plus overnight refrigeration)

Smoothie with Spinach, Pineapple, and Flaxseed

Ingredients:

1 cup spinach

1/2 cup pineapple chunks

1/2 banana

1 cup almond milk

1 tbsp flaxseed

Preparation:

1. Blend spinach, pineapple, banana, almond milk, and flaxseed until smooth.

2. Serve immediately.

Nutritional Value:

Calories: 250

Protein: 4g

Fat: 8g

Carbohydrates: 45g

Fiber: 7g   **Cooking Time: 5 minutes**

Scrambled Eggs with Tomatoes and Kale

Ingredients:

2 large eggs

1/2 cup kale, chopped

1/2 tomato, diced

1 tbsp olive oil

Salt and pepper to taste

Preparation:

1. Whisk eggs with salt and pepper.

2. Heat olive oil in a pan over medium heat.

3. Add tomatoes and kale, and cook until kale is wilted.

4. Pour in eggs and scramble until cooked through.

Nutritional Value:

Calories: 200

Protein: 12g

Fat: 16g

Carbohydrates: 6g

Fiber: 2g   **Cooking Time: 10 minutes**

Oatmeal with Almond Butter and Banana

Ingredients:

1/2 cup rolled oats

1 cup almond milk

1 tbsp almond butter

1/2 banana, sliced

1 tsp honey

1/4 tsp cinnamon

Preparation:

1. Cook rolled oats with almond milk according to package instructions.

2. Stir in almond butter.

3. Top with banana slices, honey, and cinnamon.

Nutritional Value:

Calories: 350

Protein: 10g

Fat: 14g

Carbohydrates: 48g

Fiber: 7g   **Cooking Time: 10 minutes**

Cottage Cheese with Pineapple and Chia Seeds

Ingredients:

1 cup cottage cheese (low-fat)

1/2 cup pineapple chunks

1 tbsp chia seeds

Preparation:

1. Combine cottage cheese, pineapple chunks, and chia seeds in a bowl.

2. Mix well and serve.

Nutritional Value:

Calories: 220

Protein: 20g

Fat: 5g

Carbohydrates: 22g

Fiber: 4g   **Cooking Time: 5 minutes**

Smoothie with Kale, Mango, and Chia Seeds

Ingredients:

1 cup kale

1/2 cup mango chunks

1/2 banana

1 cup almond milk

1 tbsp chia seeds

Preparation:

1. Blend kale, mango, banana, almond milk, and chia seeds until smooth.

2. Serve immediately.

Nutritional Value:

Calories: 260

Protein: 5g

Fat: 9g

Carbohydrates: 45g

Fiber: 7g   **Cooking Time: 5 minutes**

Whole Grain Waffles with Berries

Ingredients:

1 cup whole grain waffle mix

3/4 cup water

1/2 cup fresh berries

1 tbsp honey

Preparation:

1. Mix waffle mix and water until smooth.

2. Pour batter into a preheated waffle iron and cook until golden brown.

3. Top with fresh berries and honey.

Nutritional Value:

Calories: 320

Protein: 8g

Fat: 6g

Carbohydrates: 60g

Fiber: 10g   **Cooking Time: 15 minutes**

Smoothie with Spinach, Pineapple, and Flaxseed

Ingredients:

1 cup spinach

1/2 cup pineapple chunks

1/2 banana

1 cup almond milk

1 tbsp flaxseed

Preparation:

1. Blend spinach, pineapple, banana, almond milk, and flaxseed until smooth.

2. Serve immediately.

Nutritional Value:

Calories: 250

Protein: 4g

Fat: 8g

Carbohydrates: 45g

Fiber: 7g   **Cooking Time: 5 minutes**

Lunch:

Quinoa Salad with Chickpeas and Veggies

Ingredients:

1 cup cooked quinoa

1/2 cup chickpeas, rinsed and drained

1/2 cup cherry tomatoes, halved

1/4 cup cucumber, diced

1/4 cup red bell pepper, diced

2 tbsp olive oil

1 tbsp lemon juice

Salt and pepper to taste

Preparation:

1. Combine quinoa, chickpeas, cherry tomatoes, cucumber, and red bell pepper in a bowl.

2. Drizzle with olive oil and lemon juice.

3. Season with salt and pepper, then toss to mix.

Nutritional Value:

Calories: 350

Protein: 12g

Fat: 14g

Carbohydrates: 45g

Fiber: 10g   **Cooking Time: 15 minutes**

Lentil Soup with Spinach

Ingredients:

1 cup lentils, rinsed

4 cups vegetable broth

1 cup spinach, chopped

1 carrot, diced

1 celery stalk, diced

1 onion, chopped

2 garlic cloves, minced

1 tbsp olive oil

1 tsp cumin

Salt and pepper to taste

Preparation:

1. Heat olive oil in a pot over medium heat.

2. Sauté onion, carrot, celery, and garlic until softened.

3. Add lentils, vegetable broth, cumin, salt, and pepper.

4. Bring to a boil, then reduce heat and simmer for 20 minutes.

5. Stir in spinach and cook for another 5 minutes.

Nutritional Value:

Calories: 250

Protein: 15g

Fat: 5g

Carbohydrates: 40g

Fiber: 16g

Cooking Time: 30 minutes

Grilled Chicken and Avocado Salad

Ingredients:

1 grilled chicken breast, sliced

4 cups mixed greens

1/2 avocado, sliced

1/2 cup cherry tomatoes, halved

1/4 cup red onion, sliced

2 tbsp olive oil

1 tbsp balsamic vinegar

Salt and pepper to taste

Preparation:

1. Arrange mixed greens, avocado, cherry tomatoes, and red onion on a plate.

2. Top with grilled chicken slices.

3. Drizzle with olive oil and balsamic vinegar.

4. Season with salt and pepper.

Nutritional Value:

Calories: 400

Protein: 35g

Fat: 25g

Carbohydrates: 15g

Fiber: 7g   **Cooking Time: 15 minutes**

Turkey and Avocado Wrap

Ingredients:

1 whole wheat tortilla

4 oz sliced turkey breast

1/2 avocado, mashed

1/4 cup spinach leaves

1/4 cup shredded carrots

1 tbsp hummus

Preparation:

1. Spread hummus on the tortilla.

2. Layer with turkey, avocado, spinach, and carrots.

3. Roll up the tortilla tightly.

Nutritional Value:

Calories: 350

Protein: 25g

Fat: 18g

Carbohydrates: 30g

Fiber: 8g

Cooking Time: 10 minutes

Black Bean and Quinoa Bowl

Ingredients:

1 cup cooked quinoa

1/2 cup black beans, rinsed and drained

1/2 cup corn kernels

1/2 cup cherry tomatoes, halved

1/4 cup red onion, diced

1/4 cup cilantro, chopped

2 tbsp olive oil

1 tbsp lime juice

Salt and pepper to taste

Preparation:

1. Combine quinoa, black beans, corn, cherry tomatoes, red onion, and cilantro in a bowl.

2. Drizzle with olive oil and lime juice.

3. Season with salt and pepper, then toss to mix.

Nutritional Value:

Calories: 400

Protein: 15g

Fat: 14g

Carbohydrates: 55g

Fiber: 12g

Cooking Time: 15 minutes

Baked Salmon with Asparagus

Ingredients:

1 salmon fillet (about 6 oz)

1 bunch asparagus, trimmed

1 tbsp olive oil

1 lemon, sliced

Salt and pepper to taste

Preparation:

1. Preheat oven to 375°F (190°C).

2. Place salmon fillet on a baking sheet lined with parchment paper.

3. Arrange asparagus around the salmon.

4. Drizzle olive oil over the salmon and asparagus.

5. Top with lemon slices and season with salt and pepper.

6. Bake for 20-25 minutes until the salmon is cooked through.

Nutritional Value:

Calories: 350

Protein: 30g

Fat: 20g

Carbohydrates: 8g

Fiber: 4g

Cooking Time: 30 minutes

Chickpea and Avocado Salad

Ingredients:

1 cup chickpeas, rinsed and drained

1/2 avocado, diced

1/2 cup cherry tomatoes, halved

1/4 cup cucumber, diced

2 tbsp olive oil

1 tbsp lemon juice

Salt and pepper to taste

Preparation:

1. Combine chickpeas, avocado, cherry tomatoes, and cucumber in a bowl.

2. Drizzle with olive oil and lemon juice.

3. Season with salt and pepper, then toss to mix.

Nutritional Value:

Calories: 300

Protein: 10g

Fat: 20g

Carbohydrates: 25g

Fiber: 10g   **Cooking Time: 10 minutes**

Turkey Chili

Ingredients:

1 lb ground turkey

1 can (15 oz) kidney beans, rinsed and drained

1 can (15 oz) diced tomatoes

1 onion, chopped

2 garlic cloves, minced

1 red bell pepper, diced

1 tbsp olive oil

1 tbsp chili powder

1 tsp cumin

Salt and pepper to taste

Preparation:

1. Heat olive oil in a pot over medium heat.

2. Add onion, garlic, and bell pepper, and sauté until softened.

3. Add ground turkey and cook until browned.

4. Stir in kidney beans, diced tomatoes, chili powder, cumin, salt, and pepper.

5. Simmer for 20-25 minutes.

Nutritional Value:

Calories: 350

Protein: 30g

Fat: 10g

Carbohydrates: 35g

Fiber: 12g   **Cooking Time: 30 minutes**

Spinach and Chickpea Salad

Ingredients:

4 cups spinach leaves

1 cup chickpeas, rinsed and drained

1/2 red bell pepper, diced

1/4 cup red onion, sliced

2 tbsp olive oil

1 tbsp balsamic vinegar

Salt and pepper to taste

Preparation:

1. Arrange spinach leaves, chickpeas, red bell pepper, and red onion on a plate.

2. Drizzle with olive oil and balsamic vinegar.

3. Season with salt and pepper.

Nutritional Value:

Calories: 250

Protein: 10g

Fat: 14g

Carbohydrates: 25g

Fiber: 10g   **Cooking Time: 10 minutes**

Grilled Shrimp with Quinoa and Veggies

Ingredients:

1 cup cooked quinoa

8-10 large shrimp, peeled and deveined

1/2 cup cherry tomatoes, halved

1/2 cup bell pepper, diced

2 tbsp olive oil

1 tbsp lemon juice

Salt and pepper to taste

Preparation:

1. Heat olive oil in a pan over medium heat.

2. Add shrimp and cook until pink and opaque, about 2-3 minutes per side.

3. Combine cooked quinoa, cherry tomatoes, and bell pepper in a bowl.

4. Drizzle with olive oil and lemon juice.

5. Season with salt and pepper, then toss to mix.

6. Serve shrimp over quinoa and veggies.

Nutritional Value:

Calories: 350

Protein: 25g

Fat: 14g

Carbohydrates: 30g

Fiber: 8g   **Cooking Time: 20 minutes**

Veggie and Hummus Wrap

Ingredients:

1 whole wheat tortilla

1/4 cup hummus

1/4 cup shredded carrots

1/4 cup cucumber, sliced

1/4 cup bell pepper, sliced

1/4 cup spinach leaves

Preparation:

1. Spread hummus on the tortilla.

2. Layer with shredded carrots, cucumber, bell pepper, and spinach.

3. Roll up the tortilla tightly.

Nutritional Value:

Calories: 250

Protein: 8g

Fat: 10g

Carbohydrates: 35g

Fiber: 10g   **Cooking Time: 10 minutes**

Grilled Chicken and Veggie Skewers

Ingredients:

1 chicken breast, cut into cubes

1 zucchini, sliced

1 bell pepper, cut into chunks

1 red onion, cut into chunks

2 tbsp olive oil

1 tbsp lemon juice

Salt and pepper to taste

Preparation:

1. Preheat grill to medium-high heat.

2. Thread chicken, zucchini, bell pepper, and red onion onto skewers.

3. Drizzle with olive oil and lemon juice.

4. Season with salt and pepper.

5. Grill for 10-12 minutes, turning occasionally, until chicken is cooked through.

Nutritional Value:

Calories: 300

Protein: 25g

Fat: 15g

Carbohydrates: 10g

Fiber: 3g   **Cooking Time: 20 minutes**

Sweet Potato and Black Bean Bowl

Ingredients:

1 sweet potato, diced

1/2 cup black beans, rinsed and drained

1/2 avocado, diced

1/4 cup red onion, diced

2 tbsp olive oil

1 tbsp lime juice

Salt and pepper to taste

Preparation:

1. Preheat oven to 400°F (200°C).

2. Toss sweet potato with 1 tbsp olive oil, salt, and pepper.

3. Spread on a baking sheet and roast for 25-30 minutes until tender.

4. Combine roasted sweet potato, black beans, avocado, and red onion in a bowl.

5. Drizzle with remaining olive oil and lime juice.

6. Season with salt and pepper, then toss to mix.

Nutritional Value:

Calories: 350

Protein: 10g

Fat: 18g

Carbohydrates: 45g

Fiber: 15g   **Cooking Time: 40 minutes**

Tuna Salad with Mixed Greens

Ingredients:

1 can (5 oz) tuna in water, drained

4 cups mixed greens

1/2 avocado, diced

1/2 cup cherry tomatoes, halved

1/4 cup red onion, sliced

2 tbsp olive oil

1 tbsp lemon juice

Salt and pepper to taste

Preparation:

1. Arrange mixed greens, avocado, cherry tomatoes, and red onion on a plate.

2. Top with tuna.

3. Drizzle with olive oil and lemon juice.

4. Season with salt and pepper.

Nutritional Value:

Calories: 300

Protein: 25g

Fat: 18g

Carbohydrates: 10g

Fiber: 5g

Cooking Time: 10 minutes

Veggie Stir-Fry with Tofu

Ingredients:

1 cup tofu, cubed

1 cup broccoli florets

1/2 cup bell pepper, sliced

1/2 cup snap peas

1 carrot, sliced

2 tbsp soy sauce (low-sodium)

1 tbsp olive oil

1 garlic clove, minced

1 tsp ginger, grated

1 tsp sesame oil

Preparation:

1. Heat olive oil in a pan over medium-high heat.

2. Add tofu and cook until golden brown, then remove from the pan.

3. Add garlic, ginger, broccoli, bell pepper, snap peas, and carrot to the pan.

4. Stir-fry for 5-7 minutes until vegetables are tender-crisp.

5. Return tofu to the pan.

6. Add soy sauce and sesame oil, and stir to combine.

Nutritional Value:

Calories: 250

Protein: 15g

Fat: 14g

Carbohydrates: 20g

Fiber: 6g   **Cooking Time: 20 minutes**

Dinner:

Baked Cod with Vegetables

Ingredients:

1 cod fillet (6 oz)

1 zucchini, sliced

1 bell pepper, sliced

1 red onion, sliced

1 tbsp olive oil

1 lemon, sliced

1 tsp dried thyme

Salt and pepper to taste

Preparation:

1. Preheat oven to 375°F (190°C).

2. Place cod fillet on a baking sheet lined with parchment paper.

3. Arrange zucchini, bell pepper, and red onion around the cod.

4. Drizzle with olive oil, top with lemon slices, and season with thyme, salt, and pepper.

5. Bake for 20-25 minutes until the cod is cooked through.

Nutritional Value:

Calories: 350

Protein: 35g

Fat: 14g

Carbohydrates: 20g

Fiber: 6g   **Cooking Time: 30 minutes**

Turkey Meatballs with Zucchini Noodles

Ingredients:

1 lb ground turkey

1 egg, beaten

1/4 cup breadcrumbs

1/4 cup grated Parmesan cheese

2 garlic cloves, minced

1 tsp dried oregano

Salt and pepper to taste

2 zucchini, spiralized

1 tbsp olive oil

1 cup marinara sauce

Preparation:

1. Preheat oven to 375°F (190°C).

2. In a bowl, combine ground turkey, egg, breadcrumbs, Parmesan, garlic, oregano, salt, and pepper.

3. Form mixture into meatballs and place on a baking sheet.

4. Bake for 20 minutes until cooked through.

5. Heat olive oil in a pan over medium heat and sauté zucchini noodles for 3-4 minutes.

6. Serve meatballs over zucchini noodles with marinara sauce.

Nutritional Value:

Calories: 400

Protein: 35g

Fat: 20g

Carbohydrates: 20g

Fiber: 4g   **Cooking Time: 35 minutes**

Grilled Salmon with Quinoa and Spinach

Ingredients:

1 salmon fillet (6 oz)

1 cup cooked quinoa

1 cup spinach leaves

1 tbsp olive oil

1 lemon, juiced

Salt and pepper to taste

Preparation:

1. Preheat grill to medium-high heat.

2. Season salmon with olive oil, lemon juice, salt, and pepper.

3. Grill salmon for 4-5 minutes per side until cooked through.

4. Serve salmon over a bed of quinoa and spinach.

Nutritional Value:

Calories: 450

Protein: 40g

Fat: 20g

Carbohydrates: 30g

Fiber: 6g **Cooking Time: 20 minutes**

Chicken and Vegetable Stir-Fry

Ingredients:

1 chicken breast, sliced

1 cup broccoli florets

1 bell pepper, sliced

1 carrot, sliced

1/2 cup snap peas

2 tbsp soy sauce (low-sodium)

1 tbsp olive oil

1 garlic clove, minced

1 tsp ginger, grated

1 tsp sesame oil

Preparation:

1. Heat olive oil in a pan over medium-high heat.

2. Add chicken and cook until browned, then remove from the pan.

3. Add garlic, ginger, broccoli, bell pepper, carrot, and snap peas to the pan.

4. Stir-fry for 5-7 minutes until vegetables are tender-crisp.

5. Return chicken to the pan.

6. Add soy sauce and sesame oil, and stir to combine.

Nutritional Value:

Calories: 350

Protein: 30g

Fat: 14g

Carbohydrates: 20g

Fiber: 6g   **Cooking Time: 20 minutes**

Eggplant Parmesan

Ingredients:

1 large eggplant, sliced

1 cup marinara sauce

1/2 cup shredded mozzarella cheese

1/4 cup grated Parmesan cheese

1/4 cup breadcrumbs

1 egg, beaten

1 tbsp olive oil

Salt and pepper to taste

Preparation:

1. Preheat oven to 375°F (190°C).

2. Dip eggplant slices in beaten egg, then coat with breadcrumbs.

3. Heat olive oil in a pan over medium heat and fry eggplant until golden brown.

4. Place fried eggplant in a baking dish, top with marinara sauce, mozzarella, and Parmesan.

5. Bake for 20-25 minutes until cheese is melted and bubbly.

Nutritional Value:

Calories: 350

Protein: 15g

Fat: 20g

Carbohydrates: 30g

Fiber: 8g

Cooking Time: 30 minutes

Lentil and Sweet Potato Curry

Ingredients:

1 cup lentils, rinsed

1 sweet potato, diced

1 onion, chopped

2 garlic cloves, minced

1 can (15 oz) coconut milk

1 can (15 oz) diced tomatoes

2 tbsp curry powder

1 tbsp olive oil

Salt and pepper to taste

Preparation:

1. Heat olive oil in a pot over medium heat.

2. Sauté onion and garlic until softened.

3. Add lentils, sweet potato, coconut milk, diced tomatoes, curry powder, salt, and pepper.

4. Bring to a boil, then reduce heat and simmer for 25-30 minutes until lentils and sweet potato are tender.

Nutritional Value:

Calories: 400

Protein: 15g

Fat: 18g

Carbohydrates: 50g

Fiber: 15g

Cooking Time: 35 minutes

Grilled Chicken with Asparagus and Brown Rice

Ingredients:

1 chicken breast, grilled

1 cup asparagus, trimmed

1 cup cooked brown rice

1 tbsp olive oil

1 lemon, juiced

Salt and pepper to taste

Preparation:

1. Preheat grill to medium-high heat.

2. Season chicken with olive oil, lemon juice, salt, and pepper.

3. Grill chicken for 6-7 minutes per side until cooked through.

4. Sauté asparagus in a pan with olive oil, salt, and pepper for 5-7 minutes.

5. Serve grilled chicken with asparagus and brown rice.

Nutritional Value:

Calories: 450

Protein: 35g

Fat: 15g

Carbohydrates: 45g

Fiber: 6g   **Cooking Time: 30 minutes**

8. Quinoa and Black Bean Stuffed Peppers

Ingredients:

4 bell peppers, halved and seeded

1 cup cooked quinoa

1 cup black beans, rinsed and drained

1 cup corn kernels

1/2 cup diced tomatoes

1/4 cup shredded cheddar cheese

1 tbsp olive oil

1 tsp cumin

Salt and pepper to taste

Preparation:

1. Preheat oven to 375°F (190°C).

2. In a bowl, combine quinoa, black beans, corn, diced tomatoes, olive oil, cumin, salt, and pepper.

3. Stuff bell pepper halves with the mixture and place in a baking dish.

4. Top with shredded cheddar cheese.

5. Bake for 25-30 minutes until peppers are tender and cheese is melted.

Nutritional Value:

Calories: 350

Protein: 15g

Fat: 14g

Carbohydrates: 45g

Fiber: 12g   **Cooking Time: 35 minutes**

Baked Chicken with Brussels Sprouts and Sweet Potatoes

Ingredients:

1 chicken breast, cut into chunks

1 cup Brussels sprouts, halved

1 sweet potato, diced

2 tbsp olive oil

1 tsp rosemary

Salt and pepper to taste

Preparation:

1. Preheat oven to 375°F (190°C).

2. Toss chicken, Brussels sprouts, and sweet potato with olive oil, rosemary, salt, and pepper.

3. Spread on a baking sheet and bake for 25-30 minutes until chicken is cooked through and vegetables are tender.

Nutritional Value:

Calories: 400

Protein: 30g

Fat: 18g

Carbohydrates: 35g

Fiber: 8g   **Cooking Time: 35 minutes**

Shrimp and Vegetable Skewers

Ingredients:

8-10 large shrimp, peeled and deveined

1 zucchini, sliced

1 bell pepper, cut into chunks

1 red onion, cut into chunks

2 tbsp olive oil

1 lemon, juiced

Salt and pepper to taste

Preparation:

1. Preheat grill to medium-high heat.

2. Thread shrimp, zucchini, bell pepper, and red onion onto skewers.

3. Drizzle with olive oil and lemon juice.

4. Season with salt and pepper.

5. Grill for 10-12 minutes, turning occasionally, until shrimp is cooked through.

Nutritional Value:

Calories: 300

Protein: 20g

Fat: 12g

Carbohydrates: 20g

Fiber: 5g   **Cooking Time: 20 minutes**

Tofu and Vegetable Stir-Fry

Ingredients:

1 cup tofu, cubed

1 cup broccoli florets

1/2 cup bell pepper, sliced

1/2 cup snap peas

1 carrot, sliced

2 tbsp soy sauce (low-sodium)

1 tbsp olive oil

1 garlic clove, minced

1 tsp ginger, grated

1 tsp sesame oil

Preparation:

1. Heat olive oil in a pan over medium-high heat.

2. Add tofu and cook until golden brown, then remove from the pan.

3. Add garlic, ginger, broccoli, bell pepper, snap peas, and carrot to the pan.

4. Stir-fry for 5-7 minutes until vegetables are tender-crisp.

5. Return tofu to the pan.

6. Add soy sauce and sesame oil, and stir to combine.

Nutritional Value:

Calories: 250

Protein: 15g

Fat: 14g

Carbohydrates: 20g

Fiber: 6g   **Cooking Time: 20 minutes**

Baked Tilapia with Spinach and Tomatoes

Ingredients:

1 tilapia fillet (6 oz)

1 cup cherry tomatoes, halved

1 cup spinach leaves

1 tbsp olive oil

1 lemon, juiced

Salt and pepper to taste

Preparation:

1. Preheat oven to 375°F (190°C).

2. Place tilapia fillet on a baking sheet lined with parchment paper.

3. Arrange cherry tomatoes and spinach around the tilapia.

4. Drizzle with olive oil and lemon juice.

5. Season with salt and pepper.

6. Bake for 20-25 minutes until tilapia is cooked through.

Nutritional Value:

Calories: 300

Protein: 30g

Fat: 15g

Carbohydrates: 10g

Fiber: 4g   **Cooking Time: 30 minutes**

Chickpea and Vegetable Stew

Ingredients:

1 cup chickpeas, rinsed and drained

1 zucchini, diced

1 bell pepper, diced

1 carrot, sliced

1 onion, chopped

2 garlic cloves, minced

1 can (15 oz) diced tomatoes

2 cups vegetable broth

1 tbsp olive oil

1 tsp cumin

Salt and pepper to taste

Preparation:

1. Heat olive oil in a pot over medium heat.

2. Sauté onion and garlic until softened.

3. Add chickpeas, zucchini, bell pepper, carrot, diced tomatoes, vegetable broth, cumin, salt, and pepper.

4. Bring to a boil, then reduce heat and simmer for 25-30 minutes until vegetables are tender.

Nutritional Value:

Calories: 350

Protein: 12g

Fat: 12g

Carbohydrates: 50g

Fiber: 14g   **Cooking Time: 35 minutes**

Baked Chicken with Brussels Sprouts and Sweet Potatoes

Ingredients:

1 chicken breast, cut into chunks

1 cup Brussels sprouts, halved

1 sweet potato, diced

2 tbsp olive oil

1 tsp rosemary

Salt and pepper to taste

Preparation:

1. Preheat oven to 375°F (190°C).

2. Toss chicken, Brussels sprouts, and sweet potato with olive oil, rosemary, salt, and pepper.

3. Spread on a baking sheet and bake for 25-30 minutes until chicken is cooked through and vegetables are tender.

Nutritional Value:

Calories: 400

Protein: 30g

Fat: 18g

Carbohydrates: 35g

Fiber: 8g

Cooking Time: 35 minutes

Ingredients:

4 bell peppers, halved and seeded

1 cup cooked quinoa

1 cup black beans, rinsed and drained

1 cup corn kernels

1/2 cup diced tomatoes

1/4 cup shredded cheddar cheese

1 tbsp olive oil

1 tsp cumin

Salt and pepper to taste

Preparation:

1. Preheat oven to 375°F (190°C).

2. In a bowl, combine quinoa, black beans, corn, diced tomatoes, olive oil, cumin, salt, and pepper.

3. Stuff bell pepper halves with the mixture and place in a baking dish.

4. Top with shredded cheddar cheese.

5. Bake for 25-30 minutes until peppers are tender and cheese is melted.

Nutritional Value:

Calories: 350

Protein: 15g

Fat: 14g

Carbohydrates: 45g

Fiber: 12g   **Cooking Time: 35 minutes**

Snacks and Desserts:

Apple Slices with Almond Butter

Ingredients:

1 apple, sliced

2 tbsp almond butter

Preparation:

1. Core and slice the apple.

2. Serve apple slices with almond butter for dipping.

Nutritional Value:

Calories: 200

Protein: 4g

Fat: 10g

Carbohydrates: 28g

Fiber: 6g   **Cooking Time: 5 minutes**

Greek Yogurt with Berries

Ingredients:

1 cup Greek yogurt

1/2 cup mixed berries (blueberries, strawberries, raspberries)

1 tbsp honey

Preparation:

1. Spoon Greek yogurt into a bowl.

2. Top with mixed berries and drizzle with honey.

Nutritional Value:

Calories: 200

Protein: 15g

Fat: 5g

Carbohydrates: 25g

Fiber: 4g   **Cooking Time: 5 minutes**

Carrot Sticks with Hummus

Ingredients:

2 large carrots, peeled and cut into sticks

1/4 cup hummus

Preparation:

1. Cut carrots into sticks.

2. Serve carrot sticks with hummus for dipping.

Nutritional Value:

Calories: 150

Protein: 4g

Fat: 7g

Carbohydrates: 18g

Fiber: 6g

Cooking Time: 5 minutes

Chia Seed Pudding

Ingredients:

1/4 cup chia seeds

1 cup almond milk

1 tbsp maple syrup

1/2 tsp vanilla extract

Preparation:

1. In a bowl, combine chia seeds, almond milk, maple syrup, and vanilla extract.

2. Stir well and refrigerate for at least 2 hours or overnight until thickened.

Nutritional Value:

Calories: 200

Protein: 6g

Fat: 9g

Carbohydrates: 23g

Fiber: 10g

Cooking Time: 5 minutes (plus chilling time)

Avocado Toast

Ingredients:

1 slice whole-grain bread

1/2 avocado, mashed

1/2 tsp lemon juice

Salt and pepper to taste

Preparation:

1. Toast the bread.

2. Mash avocado with lemon juice, salt, and pepper.

3. Spread mashed avocado on toast.

Nutritional Value:

Calories: 200

Protein: 4g

Fat: 12g

Carbohydrates: 20g

Fiber: 7g

Cooking Time: 5 minutes

Oatmeal Energy Balls

Ingredients:

1 cup rolled oats

1/2 cup almond butter

1/4 cup honey

1/4 cup dark chocolate chips

1/4 cup flaxseeds

Preparation:

1. In a bowl, combine rolled oats, almond butter, honey, dark chocolate chips, and flaxseeds.

2. Mix until well combined.

3. Roll mixture into small balls and refrigerate for at least 30 minutes.

Nutritional Value:

Calories: 150 per ball

Protein: 4g

Fat: 8g

Carbohydrates: 18g

Fiber: 4g   **Cooking Time: 10 minutes (plus chilling time)**

Baked Sweet Potato Fries

Ingredients:

1 large sweet potato, cut into fries

1 tbsp olive oil

1/2 tsp paprika

Salt and pepper to taste

Preparation:

1. Preheat oven to 425°F (220°C).

2. Toss sweet potato fries with olive oil, paprika, salt, and pepper.

3. Spread on a baking sheet and bake for 20-25 minutes, turning halfway through.

Nutritional Value:

Calories: 200

Protein: 2g

Fat: 7g

Carbohydrates: 30g

Fiber: 4g   **Cooking Time: 30 minutes**

Cottage Cheese with Pineapple

Ingredients:

1/2 cup cottage cheese

1/2 cup pineapple chunks

Preparation:

1. Spoon cottage cheese into a bowl.

2. Top with pineapple chunks.

Nutritional Value:

Calories: 150

Protein: 12g

Fat: 5g

Carbohydrates: 15g

Fiber: 2g

Cooking Time: 5 minutes

Mixed Nuts and Dried Fruit

Ingredients:

1/4 cup mixed nuts (almonds, walnuts, cashews)

1/4 cup dried fruit (raisins, cranberries, apricots)

Preparation:

1. Combine mixed nuts and dried fruit in a bowl.

Nutritional Value:

Calories: 200

Protein: 5g

Fat: 12g

Carbohydrates: 20g

Fiber: 4g   **Cooking Time: 5 minutes**

Baked Apple Chips

Ingredients:

2 apples, thinly sliced

1 tsp cinnamon

Preparation:

1. Preheat oven to 225°F (110°C).

2. Arrange apple slices on a baking sheet lined with parchment paper.

3. Sprinkle with cinnamon.

4. Bake for 2-3 hours until crispy.

Nutritional Value:

Calories: 100

Protein: 0g

Fat: 0g

Carbohydrates: 25g

Fiber: 5g   **Cooking Time: 3 hours**

Banana Oat Cookies

Ingredients:

2 ripe bananas, mashed

1 cup rolled oats

1/4 cup dark chocolate chips

Preparation:

1. Preheat oven to 350°F (175°C).

2. In a bowl, combine mashed bananas, rolled oats, and dark chocolate chips.

3. Drop spoonfuls of the mixture onto a baking sheet.

4. Bake for 15 minutes.

Nutritional Value:

Calories: 100 per cookie

Protein: 2g

Fat: 2g

Carbohydrates: 20g

Fiber: 3g   **Cooking Time: 20 minutes**

Berry Smoothie

Ingredients:

1 cup mixed berries (frozen)

1/2 banana

1 cup almond milk

1 tbsp chia seeds

Preparation:

1. Combine mixed berries, banana, almond milk, and chia seeds in a blender.

2. Blend until smooth.

Nutritional Value:

Calories: 200

Protein: 4g

Fat: 5g

Carbohydrates: 38g

Fiber: 8g   **Cooking Time: 5 minutes**

Avocado Chocolate Mousse

Ingredients:

2 ripe avocados

1/4 cup cocoa powder

1/4 cup maple syrup

1 tsp vanilla extract

Preparation:

1. Blend avocados, cocoa powder, maple syrup, and vanilla extract until smooth.

2. Chill in the refrigerator before serving.

Nutritional Value:

Calories: 250

Protein: 3g

Fat: 18g

Carbohydrates: 24g

Fiber: 8g   **Cooking Time: 10 minutes (plus chilling time)**

Dark Chocolate Almond Clusters

Ingredients:

1 cup dark chocolate chips

1 cup almonds

Preparation:

1. Melt dark chocolate chips in a microwave-safe bowl.

2. Stir in almonds until coated.

3. Drop spoonfuls onto a baking sheet lined with parchment paper.

4. Refrigerate until set.

Nutritional Value:

Calories: 150 per cluster

Protein: 4g

Fat: 10g

Carbohydrates: 15g

Fiber: 3g

Cooking Time: 15 minutes (plus chilling time)

Frozen Yogurt Bark

Ingredients:

1 cup Greek yogurt

1/2 cup mixed berries

1 tbsp honey

Preparation:

1. Spread Greek yogurt on a baking sheet lined with parchment paper.

2. Top with mixed berries and drizzle with honey.

3. Freeze for 2 hours until firm.

4. Break into pieces and serve.

Nutritional Value:

Calories: 100 per piece

Protein: 5g

Fat: 2g

Carbohydrates: 15g

Fiber: 2g

Cooking Time: 10 minutes (plus freezing time)

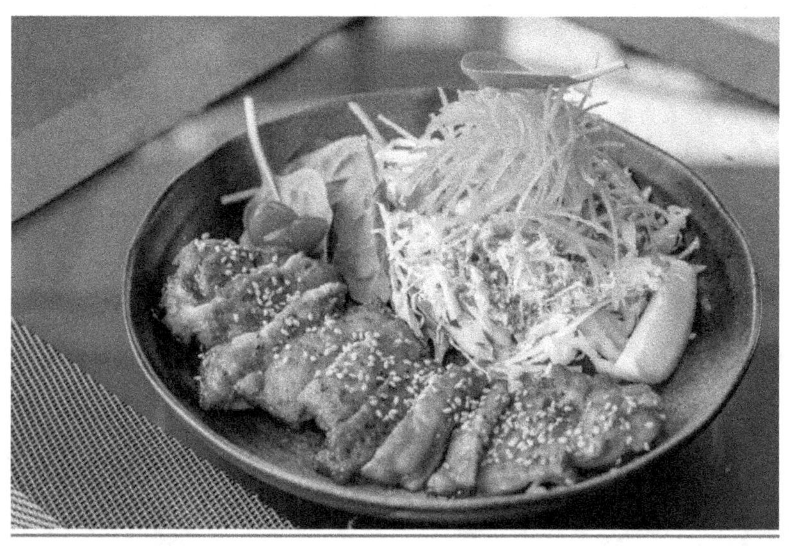

CONCLUSION

As we conclude this journey through the "Osteoarthritis Recipe Cookbook," we hope you have discovered the power of nutritious, anti-inflammatory foods in managing osteoarthritis. Each recipe, carefully crafted with wholesome ingredients, is designed to reduce inflammation, promote joint health, and enhance your overall well-being. From hearty breakfasts to satisfying lunches, delectable dinners, and tasty snacks, these meals are more than just food; they are a pathway to better health and a more vibrant life.

Living with osteoarthritis can be challenging, but adopting a diet rich in anti-inflammatory foods can make a significant difference. By incorporating these delicious and nutritious recipes into your daily routine, you are taking proactive steps to alleviate joint pain, improve mobility, and support your body's natural healing processes. The combination of fresh vegetables, lean proteins, healthy fats, and whole grains provides your body with essential nutrients to combat inflammation and strengthen your joints.

Remember, this cookbook is not just a collection of recipes; it is a guide to a healthier lifestyle. Each meal you prepare brings you one step closer to feeling better and living a more active, fulfilling life.

Embrace the joy of cooking and experimenting with these recipes, and take pride in nourishing your body with the best possible ingredients.

As you continue on this journey, know that you have the power to make positive changes in your life. Your dedication to improving your health through mindful eating is commendable. Stay motivated, stay inspired, and keep exploring new ways to incorporate these principles into your daily life. By making these recipes a part of your routine, you are investing in your future and taking control of your health.

Adopt this diet, adapt it to your preferences, and experience the transformative benefits it can bring. Here's to your health, happiness, and a future filled with delicious meals and pain-free days. Enjoy the journey and celebrate each step towards a healthier you!

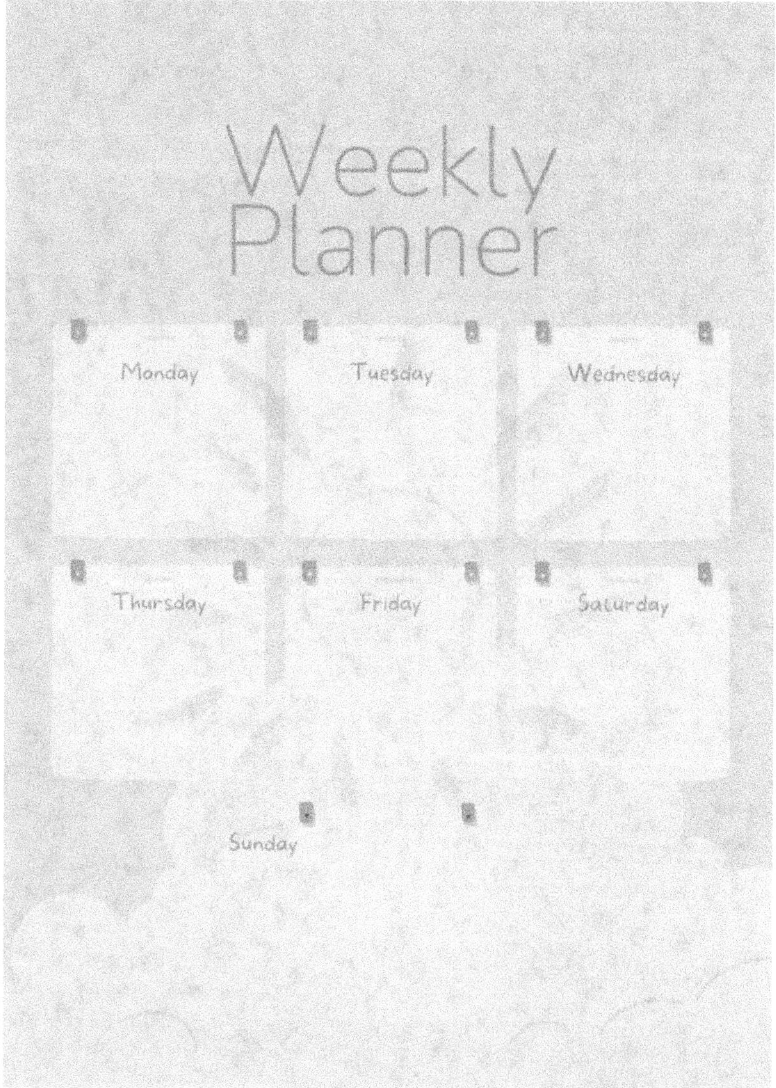
Weekly
Planner
Monday
Tuesday
Wednesday
Thursday
Friday
Saturday
Sunday

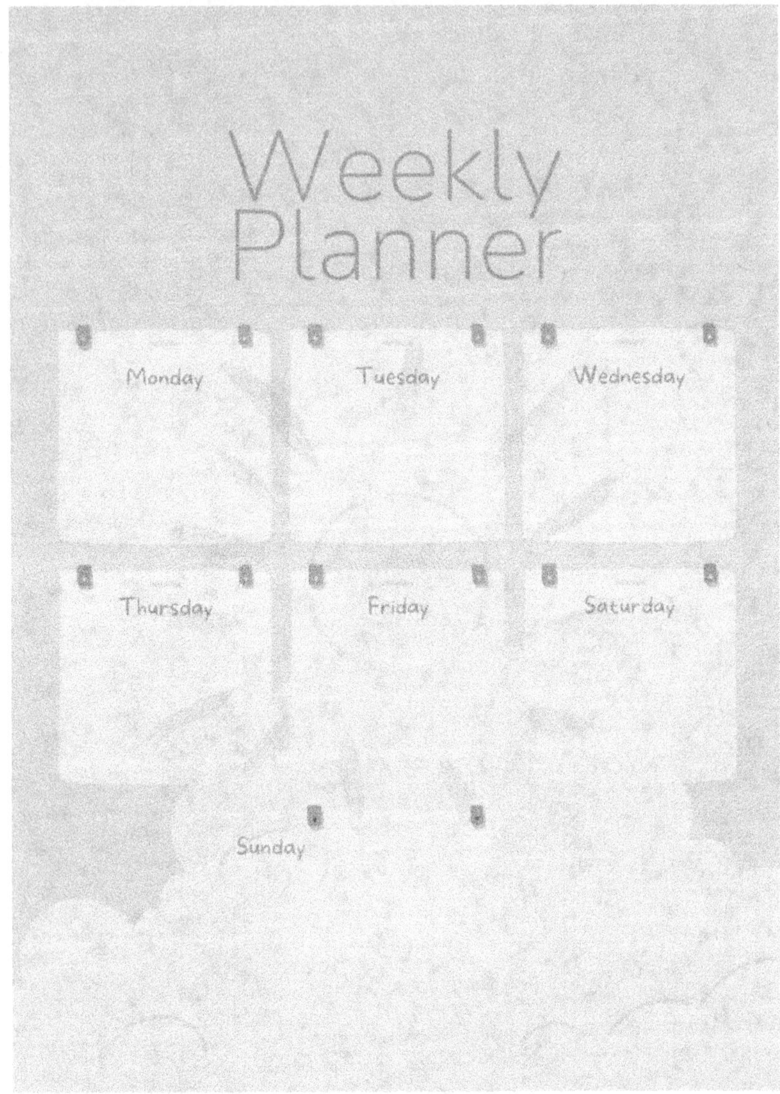
Weekly Planner
Monday
Tuesday
Wednesday
Thursday
Friday
Saturday
Sunday

Weekly Planner

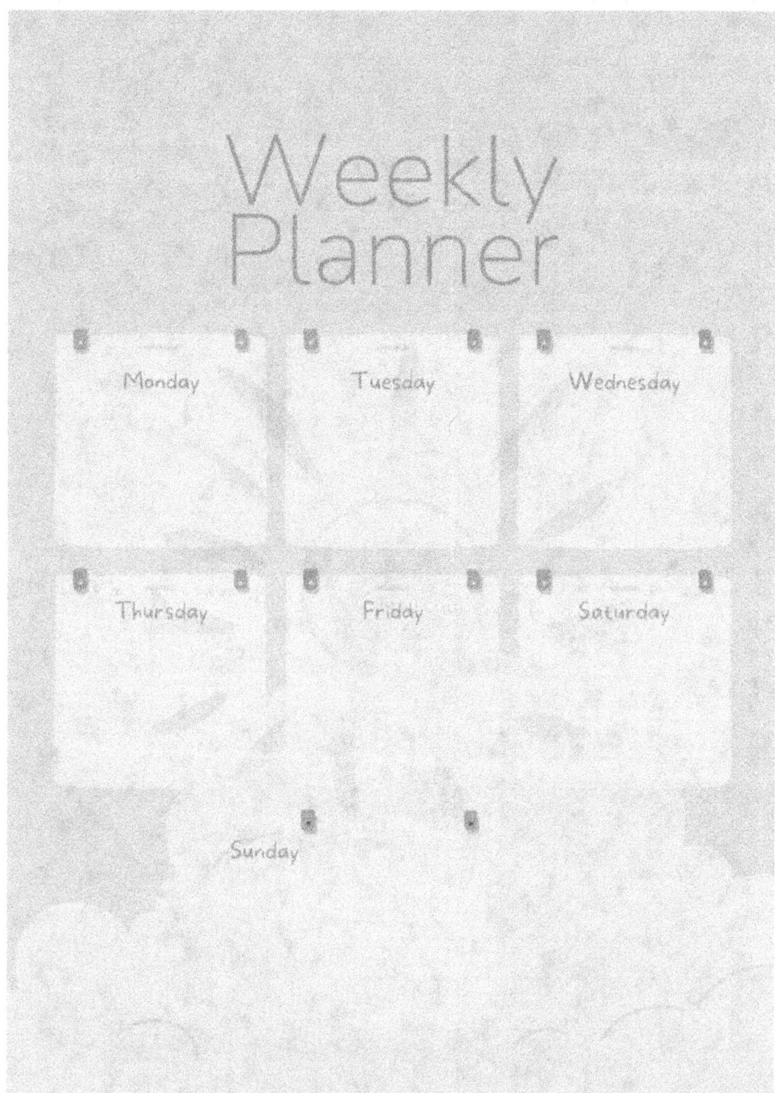

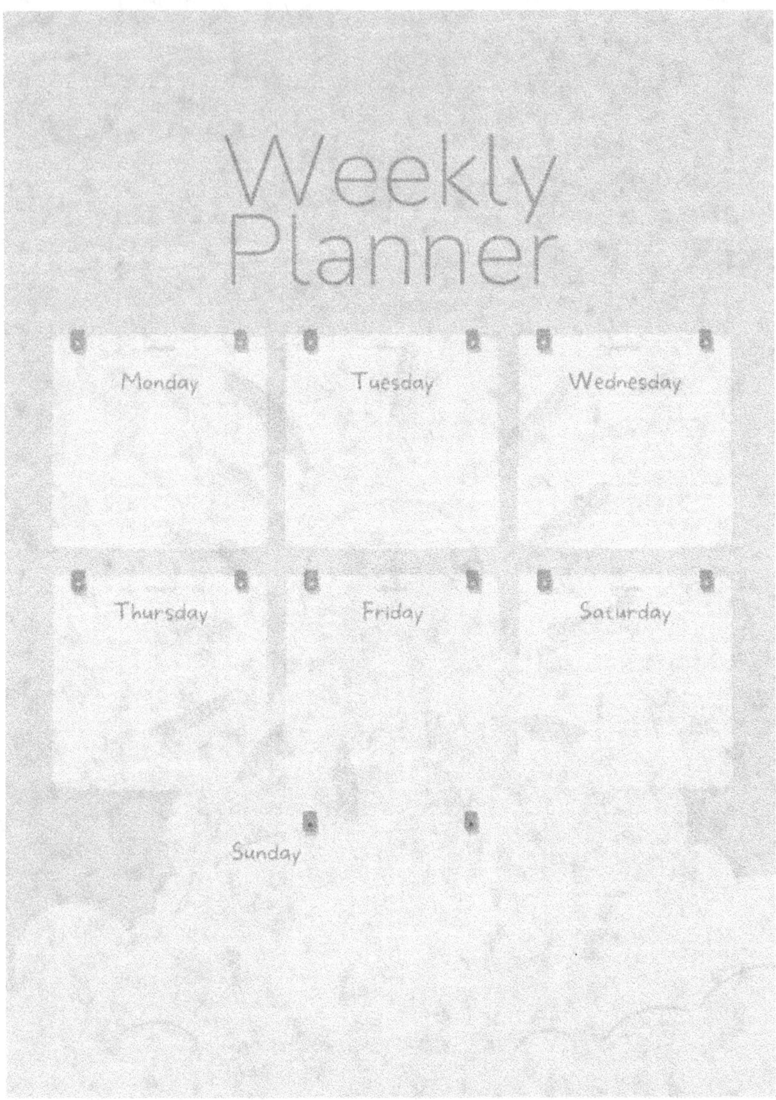

Weekly
Planner
Monday
Tuesday
Wednesday
Thursday
Friday
Saturday
Sunday

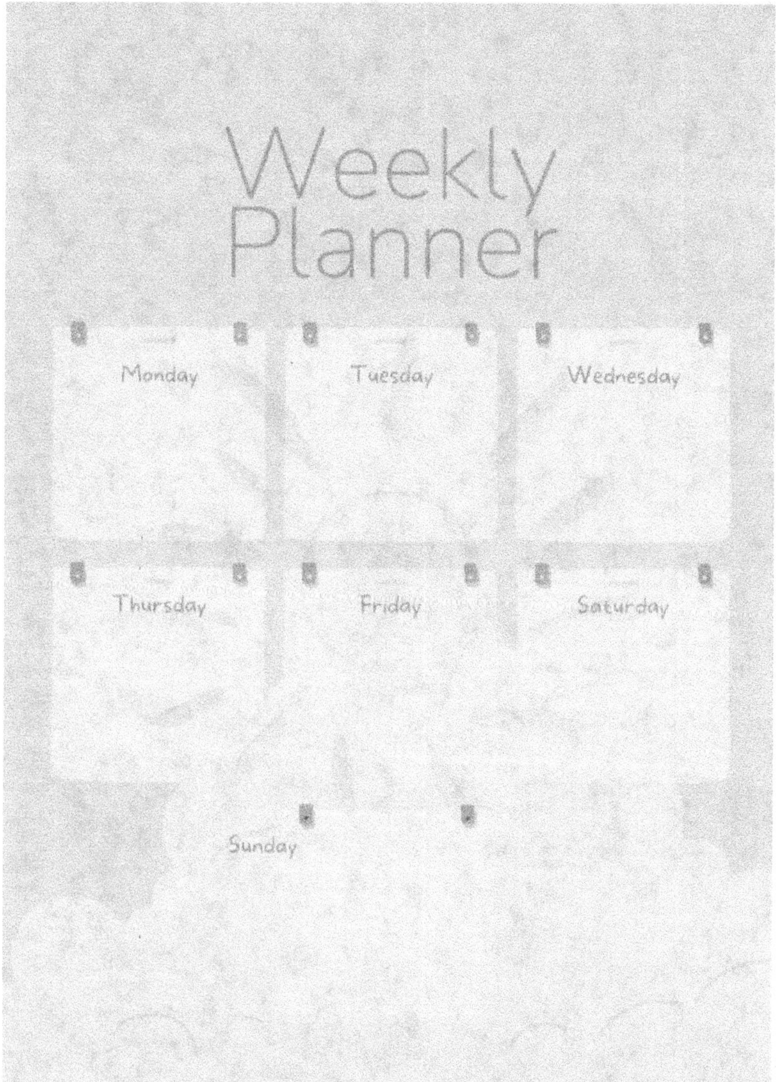

Weekly
Planner
Monday
Tuesday
Wednesday
Thursday
Friday
Saturday
Sunday

Weekly Planner

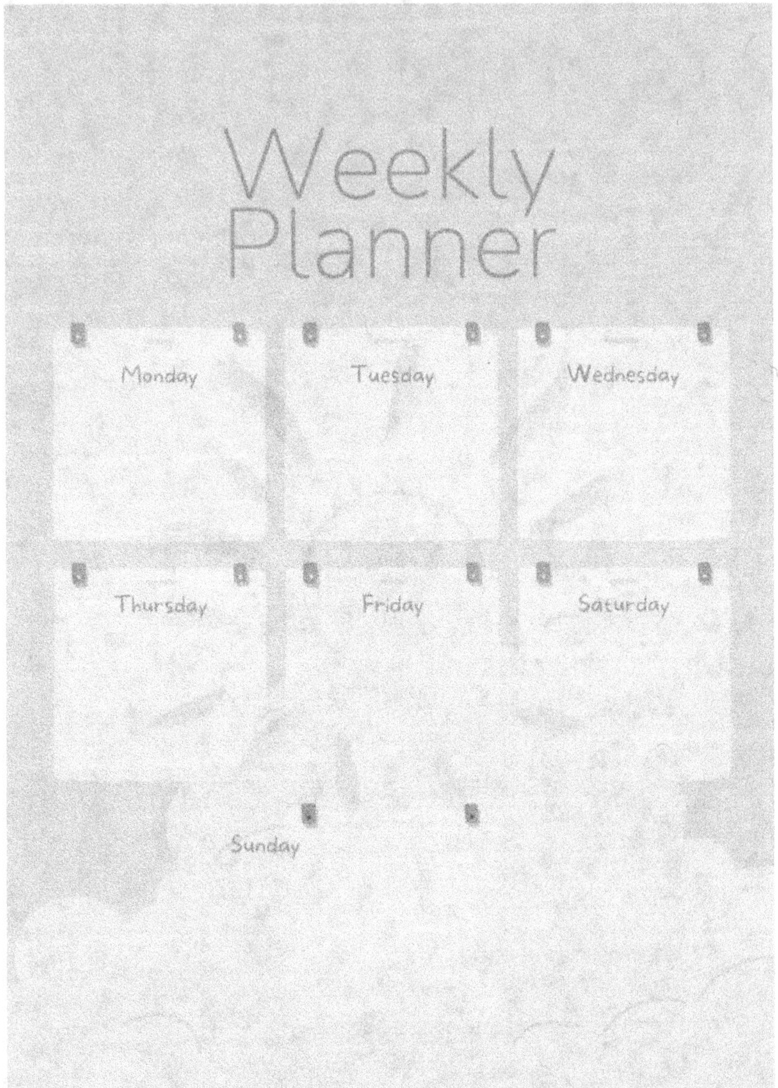

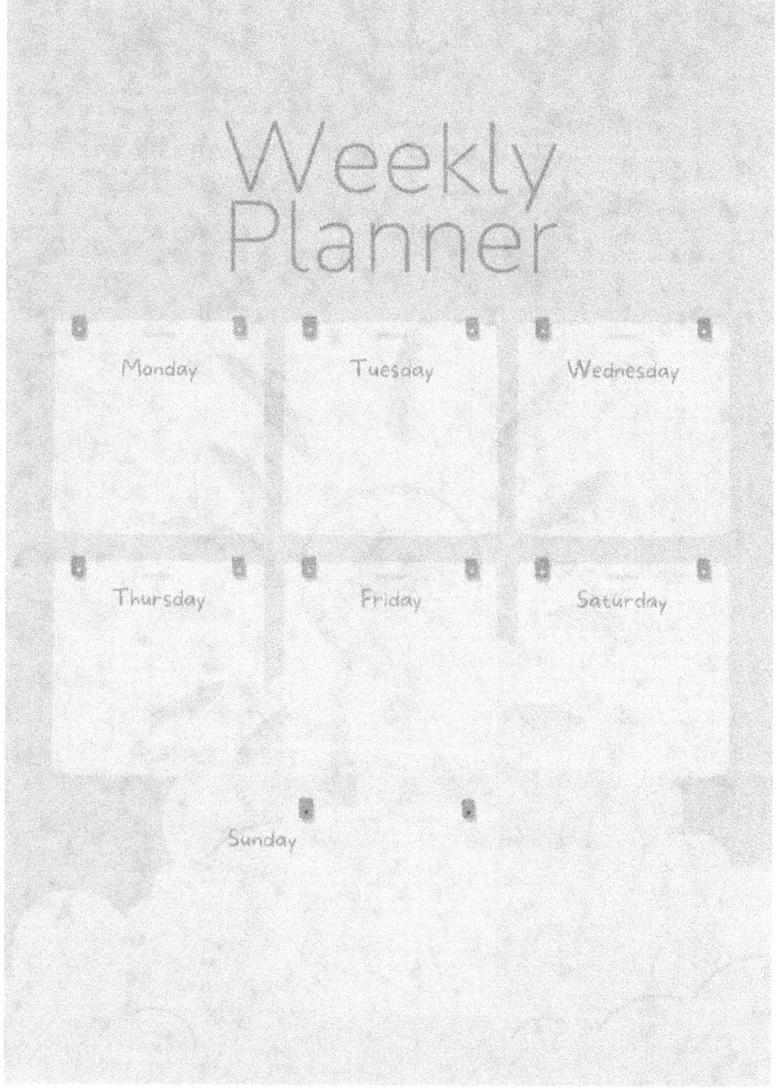

Weekly Planner
Monday
Tuesday
Wednesday
Thursday
Friday
Saturday
Sunday

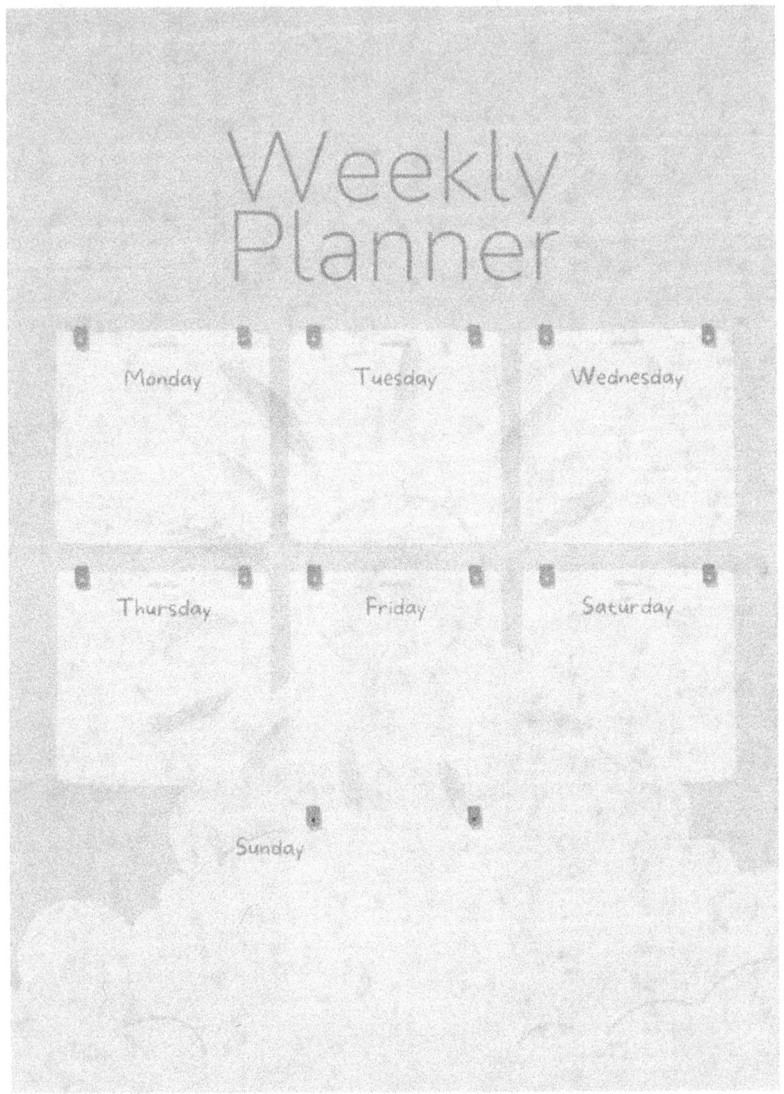

Weekly Planner
Monday
Tuesday
Wednesday
Thursday
Friday
Saturday
Sunday

Weekly Planner

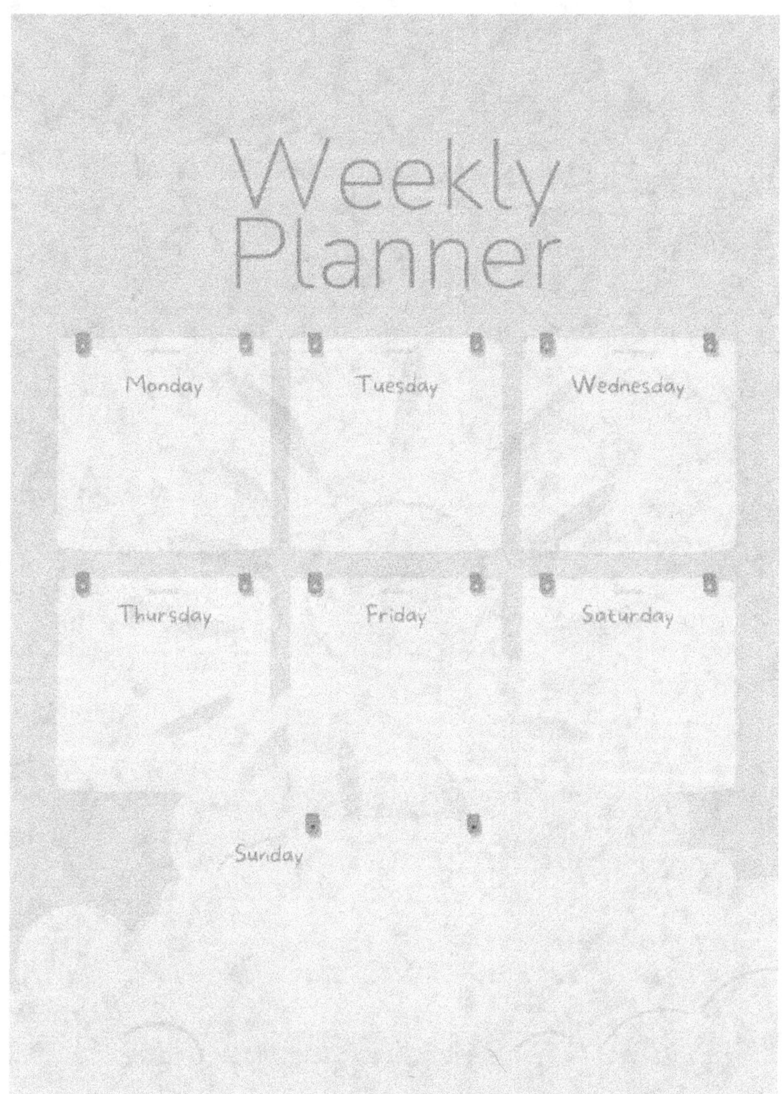

Weekly Planner

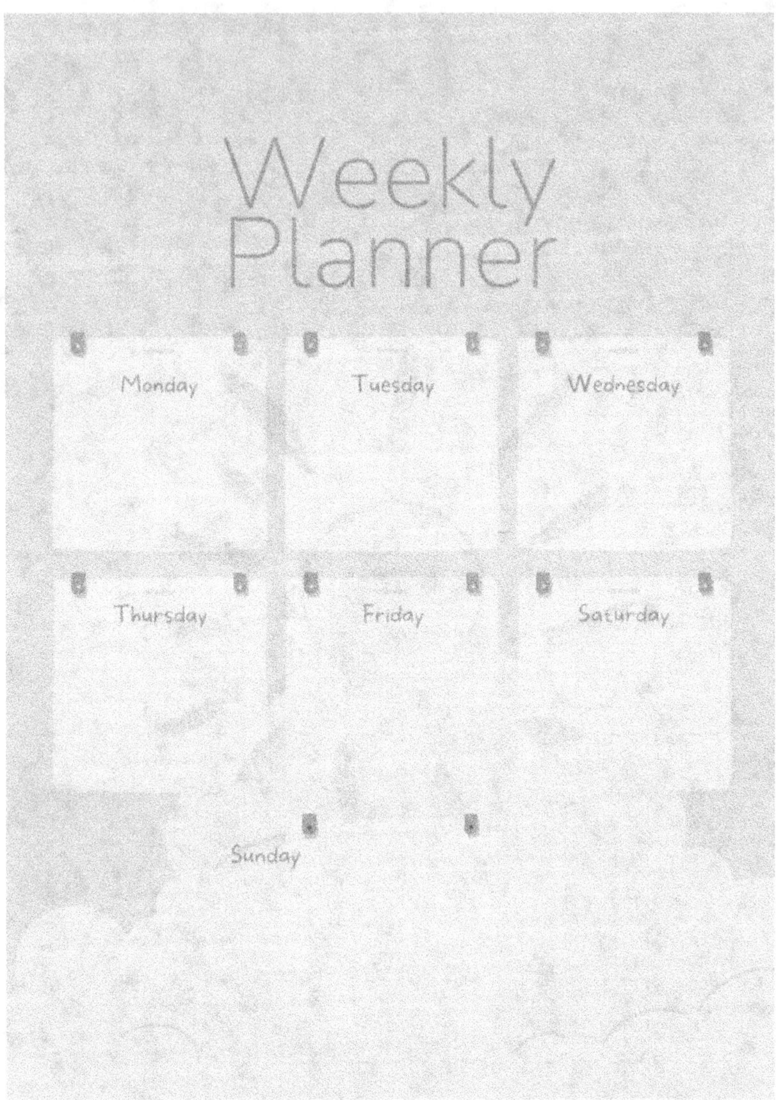

Weekly Planner

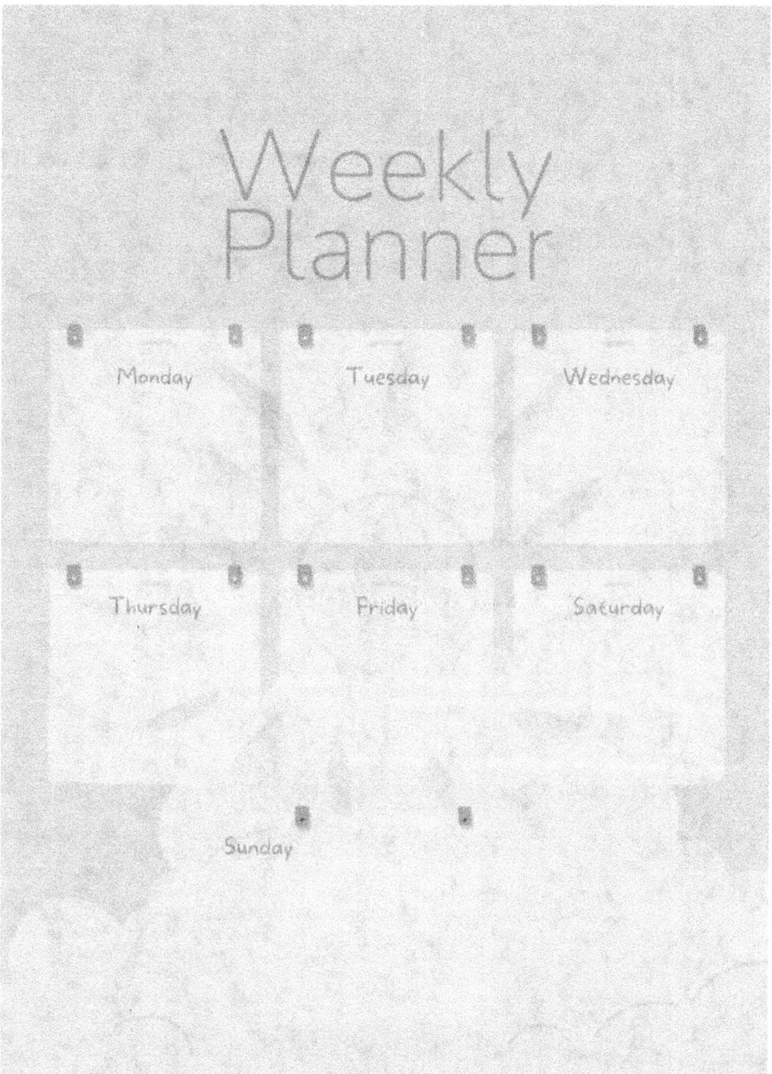

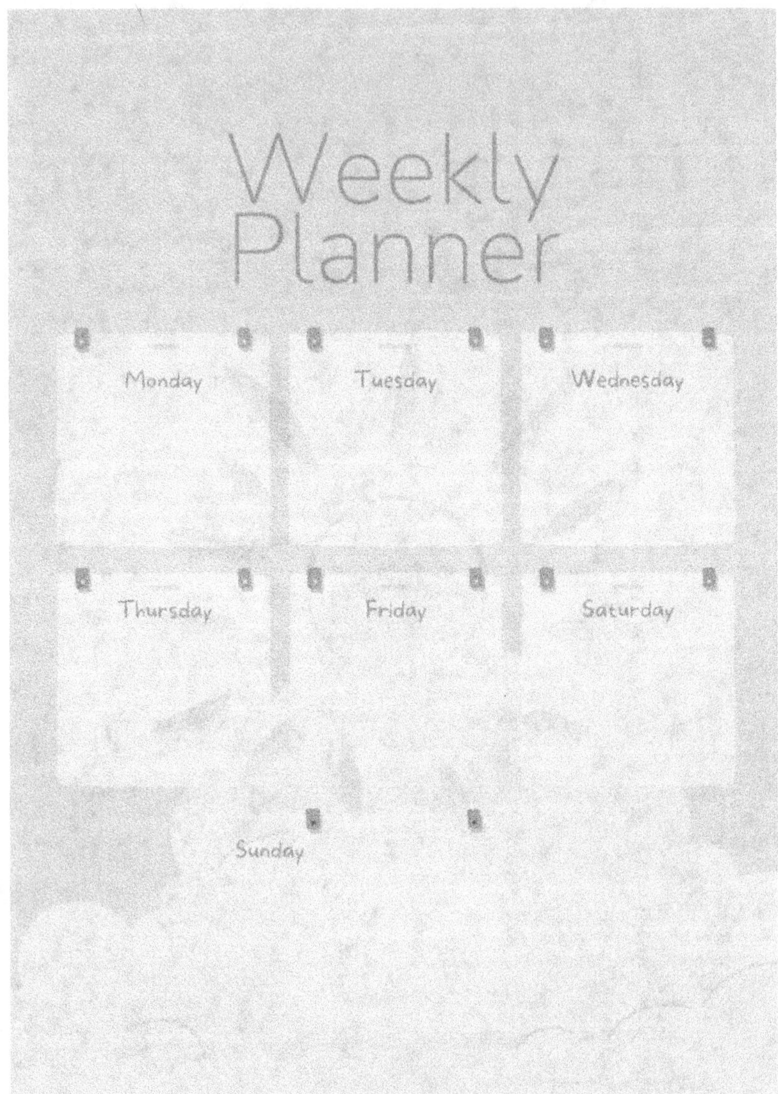
Weekly
Planner
Monday
Tuesday
Wednesday
Thursday
Friday
Saturday
Sunday

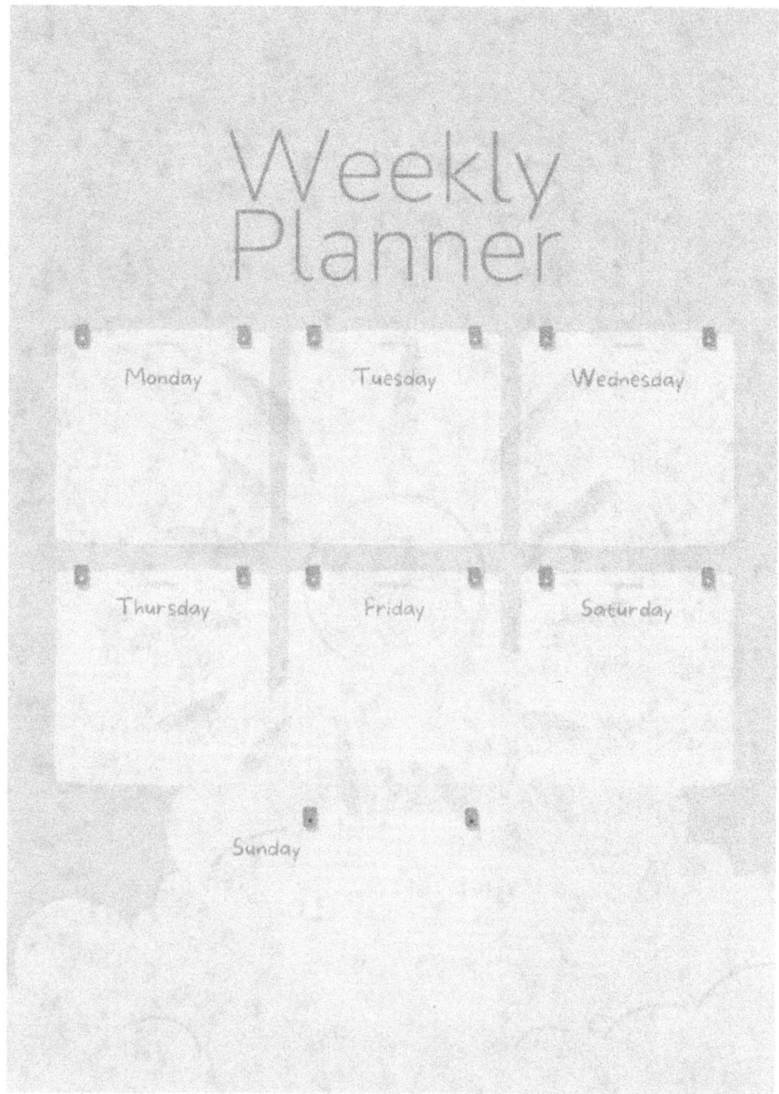

Weekly Planner
Monday
Tuesday
Wednesday
Thursday
Friday
Saturday
Sunday

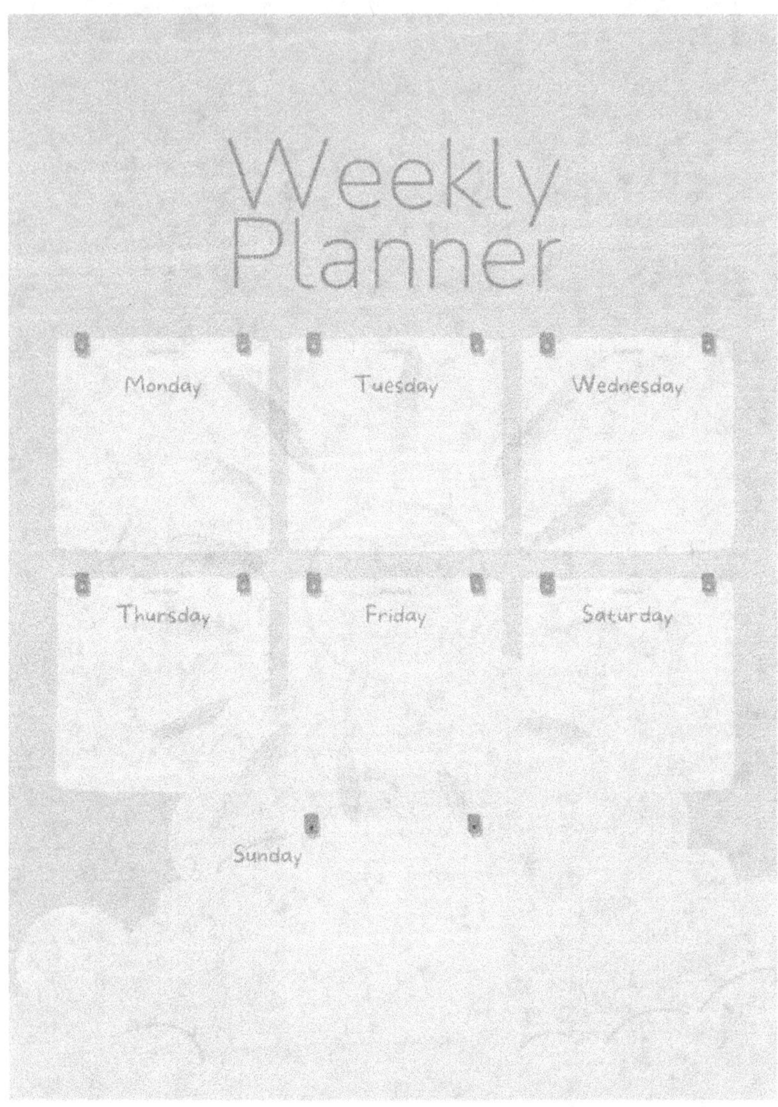

Weekly Planner
Monday
Tuesday
Wednesday
Thursday
Friday
Saturday
Sunday